The Anti Inflammatory Diet Collections

Affordable and Simple Seafood Recipes to Boost Your Health

Zac Gibson

3

Table of Contents

5

Chives Cod with Broccoli

Prep Time:
10 minutes
Cook Time:
3 hours
Serve: 4

Ingredients:

- 1-pound cod fillets
- 1 cup broccoli florets
- ½ cup vegetable stock
- 2 tablespoons tomato paste
- 2 garlic cloves, minced
- 1 red onion, minced
- ½ teaspoon rosemary, dried
- 1 tablespoon chives, chopped

Directions:

1.In your slow cooker, mix the cod with the broccoli, stock, tomato paste, and the other ingredients, toss, put the lid on and cook on Low for 3 hours.

2.Divide the mix between plates and serve.

Nutrition: 121 calories,21.6g protein, 6.7g carbohydrates, 1.2g fat, 1.8g fiber, 55mg cholesterol, 104mg sodium, 219mg potassium.

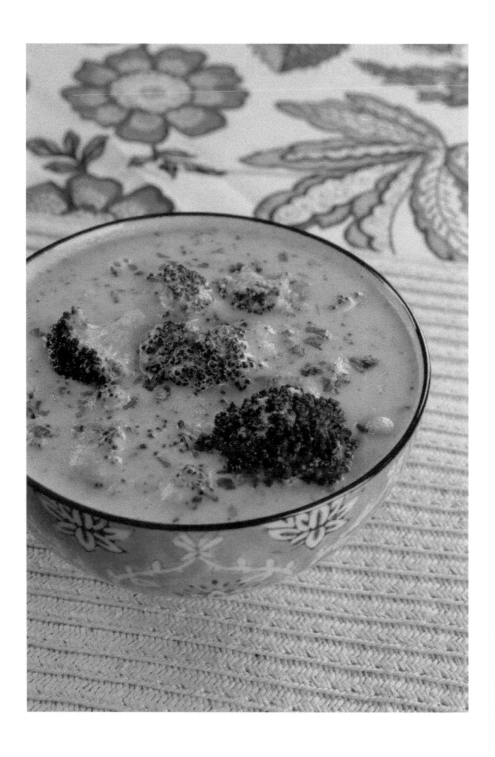

Cinnamon Trout with Cayenne Pepper

Prep Time:
5 minutes
Cook Time:
3 hours
Serve: 2

Ingredients:

- 1 pound trout fillets, boneless
- 1 tablespoon ground cinnamon
- ¼ cup chicken stock
- 2 tablespoons chili pepper, minced
- A pinch of cayenne pepper
- 1 tablespoon chives, chopped

Directions:

1.In your slow cooker, mix the trout with the cinnamon, stock, and the other ingredients, toss gently, put the lid on, and cook on Low for 3 hours.

2.Divide the mix between plates and serve with a side salad.

Nutrition: 449 calories,60.9g protein, 4.6g carbohydrates, 19.5g fat, 2.6g fiber, 168mg cholesterol, 250mg sodium, 1177mg potassium.

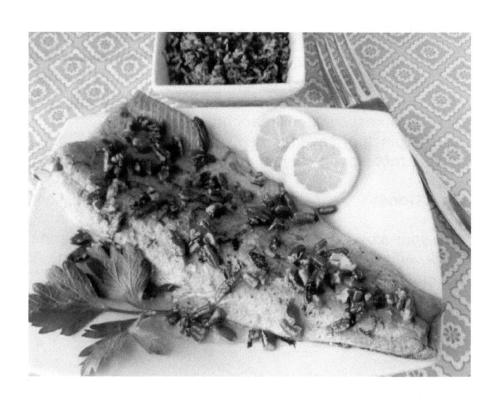

Seafood and Green Onions Mix

Prep Time:
10 minutes
Cook Time:
2 hours
Serve: 4

Ingredients:

- 1 green onions bunch, halved
- 10 tablespoons lemon juice
- 4 salmon fillets, boneless
- 2 tablespoons avocado oil

Directions:

1.Grease your Slow cooker with the oil, add salmon, top with onion, lemon juice, cover, cook on High for 2 hours, divide everything between plates and serve.

Nutrition: 255 calories,35g protein, 1.5g carbohydrates, 12.2g fat, 0.6g fiber, 78mg cholesterol, 87mg sodium, 763mg potassium.

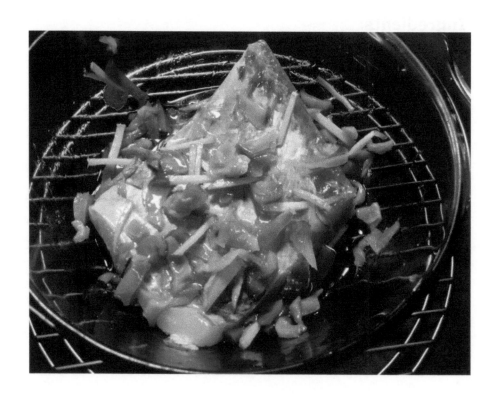

Seafood Soup

Prep Time:
10 minutes
Cook Time:
8 h & 30 m
Serve: 4

Ingredients:

- 2 cups of water
- ½ fennel bulb, chopped
- 2 sweet potatoes, cubed
- 1 yellow onion, chopped
- 2 bay leaves
- 1 tablespoon thyme, dried
- 1 celery rib, chopped
- 1 bottle clam juice
- 2 tablespoons tapioca powder
- 1 cup of coconut milk
- 1 pound salmon fillets, cubed
- 5 sea scallops, halved
- 24 shrimp, peeled and deveined
- ¼ cup parsley, chopped

Directions:

1.In your Slow cooker, mix water with fennel, potatoes, onion, bay leaves, thyme, celery, clam juice, tapioca, stir, cover, and cook on Low for 8 hours.

2.Add salmon, coconut milk, scallops, shrimp, and parsley, cook on Low for 30 minutes more, ladle chowder into bowls, and serve.

Nutrition: 547 calories,61.2g protein, 22.3g carbohydrates, 24.1g fat, 4.9g fiber, 340mg cholesterol,475mg sodium, 1458mg potassium.

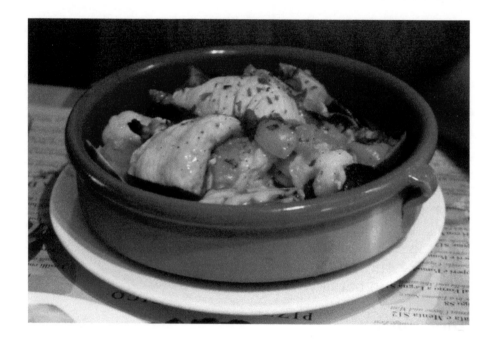

Asian Style Salmon

Prep Time:
10 minutes
Cook Time:
3 hours
Serve: 2

Ingredients:

- 2 medium salmon fillets, boneless
- 2 tablespoons maple syrup
- 16 ounces mixed broccoli and cauliflower florets
- 2 tablespoons lemon juice
- 1 teaspoon sesame seeds

Directions:

1.Put the cauliflower and broccoli florets in your Slow cooker and top with salmon fillets.

2.In a bowl, mix maple syrup with lemon juice, whisk well, pour this over salmon fillets, sprinkle sesame seeds on top, and cook on Low for 3 hours.

3.Divide everything between plates and serve.

Nutrition: 273 calories,36.9g protein, 6g carbohydrates, 12g fat, 2.7g fiber, 12mg cholesterol, 112mg sodium, 1012mg potassium.

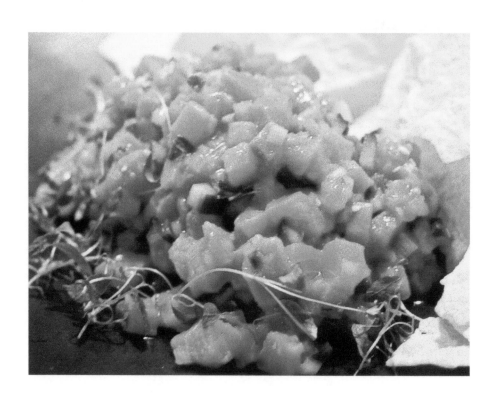

Garlic Shrimp Mix

Prep Time:
10 minutes
Cook Time:
1 h and 30 m
Serve: 4

Ingredients:

- 2 tablespoons olive oil
- 1 pound shrimp, peeled and deveined
- ¼ cup chicken stock
- 1 tablespoon garlic, minced
- 2 tablespoons parsley, chopped
- Juice of ½ lemon

Directions:

1.Put the oil in your Slow cooker, add the stock, garlic, parsley, lemon juice, and whisk well.

2.Add shrimp, stir, cover, cook on High for 1 hour and 30 minutes, divide into bowls and serve.

Nutrition: 199 calories,26.1g protein, 2.6g carbohydrates, 9g fat, 0.1g fiber, 239mg cholesterol, 326mg sodium, 212mg potassium.

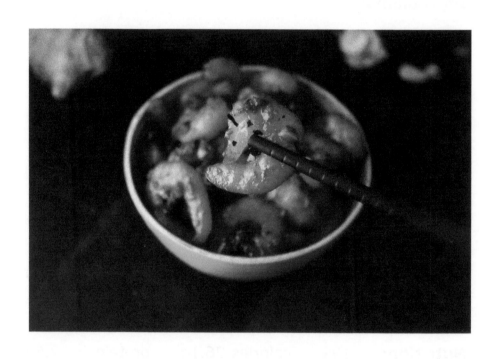

Steamed Fish

Prep Time:
10 minutes
Cook Time:
1 hour
Serve: 4

Ingredients:

- 2 tablespoons honey
- 4 salmon fillets, boneless
- 2 tablespoons soy sauce
- ¼ cup olive oil
- ¼ cup vegetable stock
- 1 small ginger piece, grated
- 6 garlic cloves, minced
- 2 tablespoons Worcestershire sauce
- 1 bunch leeks, chopped
- 1 bunch cilantro, chopped

Directions:

1.Put the oil in your slow cooker, add leeks, and top with the fish.

2.In a bowl, mix stock with ginger, honey, garlic, cilantro, and soy sauce, stir, add this over fish, cover and cook on High for 1 hour.

3.Divide fish between plates and serve with the sauce drizzled on top.

Nutrition: 397 calories,35.5g protein, 12.9g carbohydrates, 23.6g fat, 0.4g fiber, 78mg cholesterol, 624mg sodium, 761mg potassium.

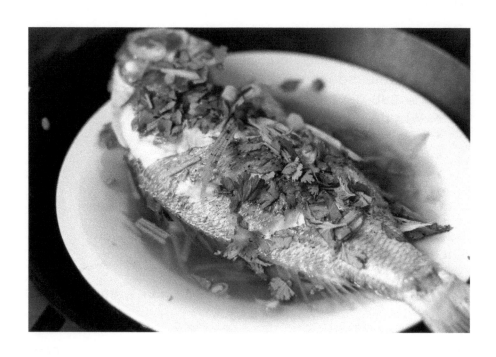

Poached Cod

Prep Time:
10 minutes
Cook Time:
4 hours
Serve: 4

Ingredients:

- 1 pound cod, boneless
- 6 garlic cloves, minced
- 1 small ginger pieces, chopped
- ½ tablespoon black peppercorns
- 1 cup pineapple juice
- 1 cup pineapple, chopped
- ¼ cup white vinegar
- 4 jalapeno peppers, chopped

Directions:

1.Put the fish in your crock.

2.Add garlic, ginger, peppercorns, pineapple juice, pineapple chunks, vinegar, and jalapenos.

3.Stir gently, cover, and cook on Low for 4 hours.

4.Divide fish between plates, top with the pineapple mix.

Nutrition: 191 calories,26.9g protein, 16.6g carbohydrates, 1.4g fat, 1.6g fiber, 6.2mg cholesterol, 460mg sodium, 484mg potassium.

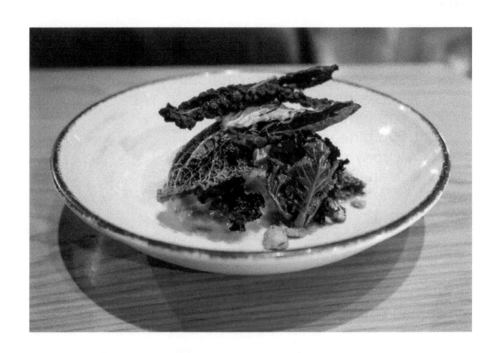

Ginger Catfish

Prep Time:
10 minutes
Cook Time:
6 hours
Serve: 4

Ingredients:

- 1 catfish, boneless and cut into 4 pieces
- 3 red chili peppers, chopped
- ½ cup of honey
- ¼ cup of water
- 1 tablespoon soy sauce
- 1 shallot, minced
- A small ginger piece, grated
- 1 tablespoon coriander, chopped

Directions:

1.Put catfish pieces in your Slow cooker.

2.Heat a pan with the coconut honey over medium-high heat and stir until it caramelizes.

3.Add soy sauce, shallot, ginger, water, and chili pepper, stir, pour over the fish, add coriander, cover and cook on Low for 6 hours.

4.Divide fish between plates and serve with the sauce from the slow cooker drizzled on top.

Nutrition: 184 calories,4.4g protein, 37.7g carbohydrates, 2.9g fat, 0.4g fiber, 18mg cholesterol, 289mg sodium, 122mg potassium.

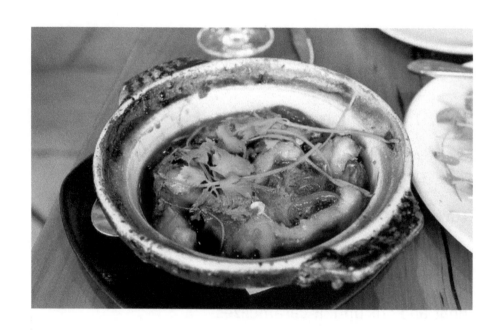

Tuna Mix

Prep Time:
10 minutes
Cook Time:
4 h & 10 m
Serve: 6

Ingredients:

- ½ pound tuna loin, cubed
- 1 garlic clove, minced
- 4 jalapeno peppers, chopped
- 1 cup olive oil
- 3 red chili peppers, chopped
- 2 teaspoons black peppercorns, ground

Directions:

1.Put the oil in your Slow cooker, add chili peppers, jalapenos, peppercorns, and garlic, whisk, cover, and cook on Low for 4 hours.

3.Add tuna, stir again, cook on High for 10 minutes more, divide between plates, and serve.

Nutrition: 366 calories,10.3g protein, 1.5g carbohydrates, 36.8g fat, 0.7g fiber, 12mg cholesterol, 265mg sodium, 170mg potassium.

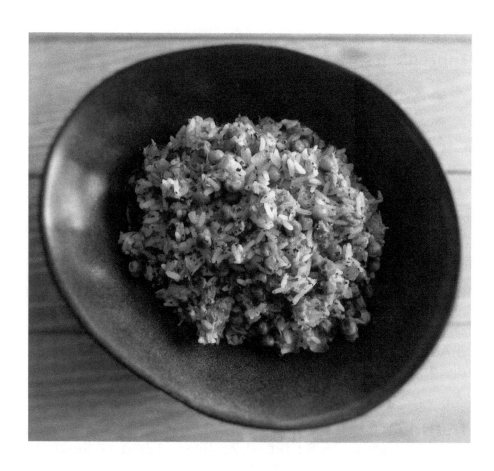

Bok Choy Sea Bass

Prep Time:
10 minutes
Cook Time:
1 h and 30 m
Serve: 4

Ingredients:

- 1 pound sea bass
- 2 scallion stalks, chopped
- 1 small ginger piece, grated
- 1 tablespoon soy sauce
- 2 cups coconut cream
- 4 bok choy stalks, chopped
- 3 jalapeno peppers, chopped

Directions:

1.Put the cream in your Slow cooker, add ginger, soy sauce, scallions, jalapenos, stir, top with the fish and bok choy, cover, and cook on High for 1 hour and 30 minutes.

2.Divide the fish mix between plates and serve.

Nutrition: 427 calories,30.3g protein, 8.6g carbohydrates, 31.7g fat, 3.4g fiber, 60mg cholesterol, 628mg sodium, 784mg potassium.

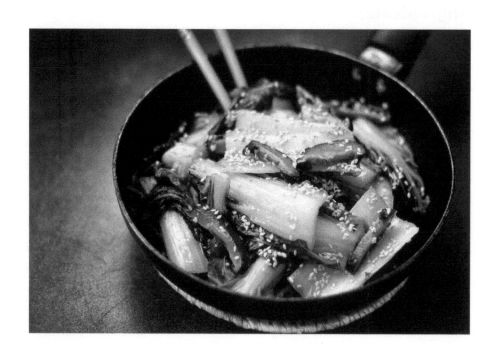

Onion Cod Fillets

Prep Time:
10 minutes
Cook Time:
2 hours
Serve: 4

Ingredients:

- 4 medium cod fillets, boneless
- ¼ teaspoon nutmeg, ground
- 1 teaspoon ginger, grated
- 1 teaspoon onion powder
- ¼ teaspoon sweet paprika
- 1 teaspoon cayenne pepper
- ½ teaspoon ground cinnamon

Directions:

1.In a bowl, mix cod fillets with nutmeg, ginger, onion powder, paprika, cayenne pepper, cinnamon, toss, transfer to your Slow cooker, cover and cook on Low for 2 hours.

2.Divide between plates and serve with a side salad.

Nutrition: 97 calories,20.2g protein, 1.4g carbohydrates, 1.2g fat, 0.4g fiber, 40mg cholesterol, 81mg sodium, 26mg potassium.

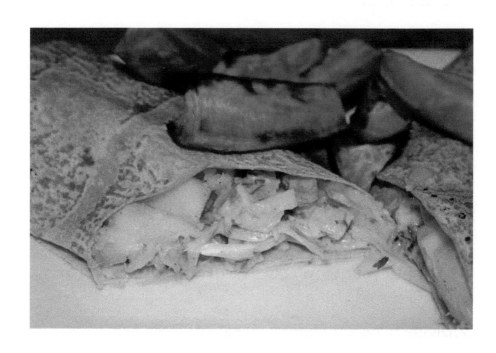

Seafood and Baby Carrots Mix

Prep Time:
10 minutes
Cook Time:
4 h & 30 m
Serve: 2

Ingredients:

- 1 small yellow onion, chopped
- 15 baby carrots
- 2 garlic cloves, minced
- 1 small green bell pepper, chopped
- 8 ounces of coconut milk
- 3 tablespoons tomato paste
- ½ teaspoon red pepper, crushed
- ¾ tablespoons curry powder
- ¾ tablespoon almond flour
- 1-pound shrimp, peeled and deveined

Directions:

1.In your food processor, mix the onion with garlic, bell pepper, tomato paste, coconut milk, red pepper, and curry powder, blend well, add to your Slow cooker, also add baby carrots, stir, cover, and cook on Low for 4 hours.

2.Add tapioca and shrimp, stir, cover, and cook on Low for 30 minutes more.

3.Divide into bowls and serve.

Nutrition: 315 calories,28.8g protein, 14.9g carbohydrates, 16.3g fat, 3.8g fiber, 239mg cholesterol, 328mg sodium, 639mg potassium.

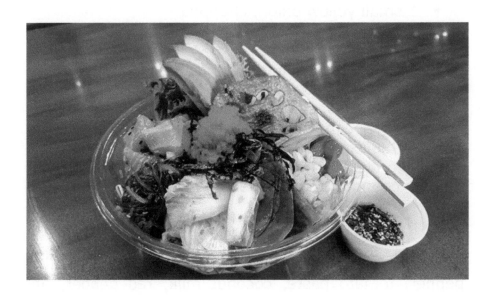

Lemon Trout with Spinach

Prep Time:
10 minutes
Cook Time:
2 hours
Serve: 4

Ingredients:

- 2 lemons, sliced
- ¼ cup chicken stock
- 2 tablespoons dill, chopped
- 12-ounce spinach
- 4 medium trout

Directions:

1.Put the stock in your Slow cooker, add the fish inside, top with lemon slices, dill, spinach, cover, and cook on High for 2 hours.

2.Divide fish, lemon, and spinach between plates and drizzle some of the juice from the slow cooker all over.

Nutrition: 150 calories,19.6g protein, 6.7g carbohydrates, 5.8g fat, 2.9g fiber, 46mg cholesterol, 160mg sodium, 8 2 54mg potassium.

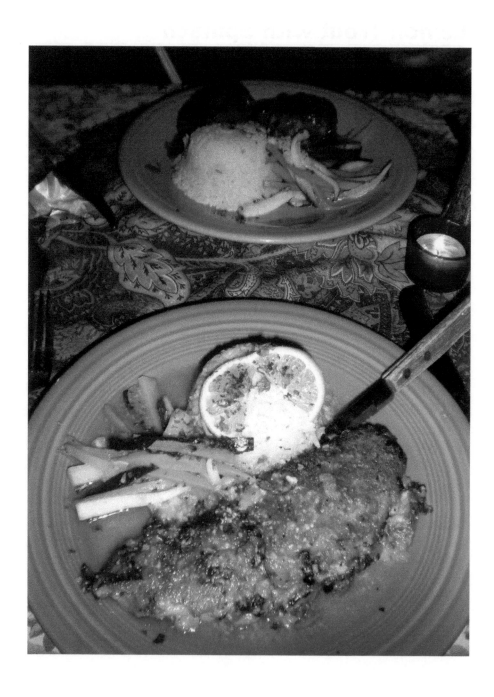

Salmon and Sweet Potatoes

Prep Time:
10 minutes
Cook Time:
25 minutes
Serve: 4

Directions:

- 4 salmon fillets, boneless
- 1 garlic cloves, minced
- 2 tablespoons olive oil
- A pinch of salt and black pepper
- 1 yellow onion, sliced
- 2 sweet potatoes, peeled and cut into wedges
- 1 tablespoon rosemary, chopped
- 1 tablespoon lime juice

Directions:

1.Grease a baking dish with the oil, arrange the salmon, garlic, onion and the other ingredients into the dish and bake everything at 380 degrees F for 25 minutes.

2.Divide the mix between plates and serve.

Nutrition: calories 260, fat 4, fiber 6, carbs 10, protein 16

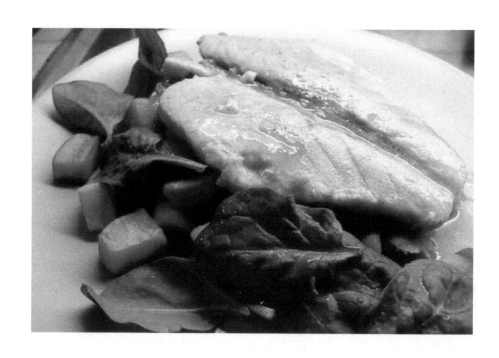

Salmon with Herbed Sauce

Prep Time:
5 minutes
Cook Time:
20 minutes
Serve: 4

Ingredients:

- 3 tablespoons olive oil
- 4 salmon fillets, boneless
- 4 garlic cloves, minced
- ¼ cup coconut cream
- 1 tablespoon parsley, chopped
- 1 tablespoon rosemary, chopped
- 1 tablespoon basil, chopped
- 1 tablespoon oregano, chopped
- 1 tablespoon pine nuts, toasted
- A pinch of salt and black pepper

Directions:

1.In a blender, combine the oil with the garlic and the other ingredients except the fish and pulse.

2.Arrange the fish in a roasting pan, add the herbed sauce on top and cook at 380 degrees F for 20 minutes.

3.Divide the mix between plates and serve.

Nutrition: calories 386, fat 26.8, fiber 1.4, carbs 3.5, protein 35.6

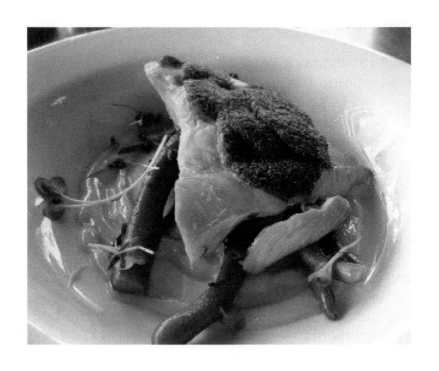

Cumin Shrimp and Beans

Prep Time:
5 minutes
Cook Time:
12 minutes
Serve: 4

Ingredients:

- 1 pound shrimp, peeled and deveined
- 2 tablespoons olive oil
- 1 teaspoon cumin, ground
- 4 green onions, chopped
- 1 cup canned black beans, drained and rinsed
- 2 tablespoons lime juice
- 1 teaspoon turmeric powder

Directions:

1.Heat a pan with the oil over medium heat, add the green onions and sauté for 2 minutes.

2.Add the shrimp and the other ingredients, toss, cook over medium heat for another 10 minutes, divide between.

Nutrition: calories 251, fat 12, fiber 2, carbs 13, protein 16

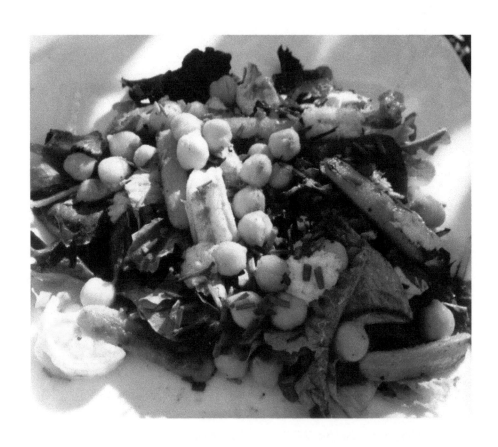

Shrimp with Spinach

Prep Time:
10 minutes
Cook Time:
10 minutes
Serve: 4

Ingredients:

- 1 pound shrimp, peeled and deveined
- 2 tablespoons olive oil
- 1 tablespoon lime juice
- 1 cup baby spinach
- A pinch of sea salt and black pepper
- 1 tablespoon chives, chopped

Directions:

1.Heat the pan with the oil over medium heat, add the shrimp and sauté for 5 minutes.

2.Add the spinach and the remaining ingredients, toss, cook the mix for another 5 minutes, divide between plates.

Nutrition: calories 206, fat 6, fiber 4, carbs 7, protein 17

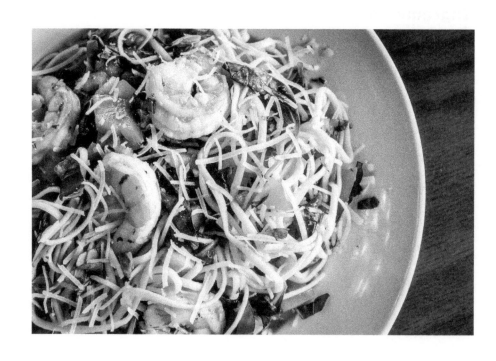

Lime Cod and Peppers

Prep Time:
10 minutes
Cook Time:
15 minutes
Serve: 4

Ingredients:

- 4 cod fillets, boneless
- 2 tablespoons olive oil
- 4 spring onions, chopped
- Juice of 1 lime
- 1 red bell pepper, cut into strips
- 1 green bell pepper, cut into strips
- 2 teaspoons parsley, chopped
- A pinch of salt and black pepper

Directions:

1.Heat a pan with the oil over medium heat, add the bell peppers and the onions and sauté for 5 minutes.

2.Add the fish and the rest of the ingredients, cook the mix for 10 minutes more, flipping the fish halfway.

3.Divide the mix between plates and serve.

Nutrition: calories 180, fat 5, fiber 1, carbs 7, protein 11

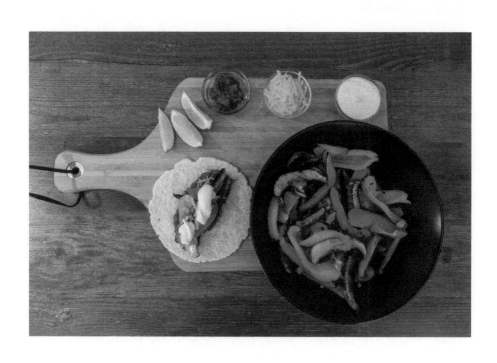

Cod Pan

Prep Time:
5 minutes
Cook Time:
20 minutes
Serve: 4

Ingredients:

- 1 pound cod fillets, boneless and cubed
- 2 tablespoons avocado oil
- 1 avocado, peeled, pitted and cubed
- 1 tomato, cubed
- 1 tablespoon lemon juice
- ¼ cup parsley, chopped
- 1 tablespoon tomato paste ½ cup veggie stock
- A pinch of sea salt and black pepper

Directions:

1.Heat a pan with the oil over medium-high heat, add the fish and cook for 3 minutes on each side.

2.Add the rest of the ingredients, cook the mix for 14 minutes more over medium heat, divide between plates and serve.

Nutrition: calories 160, fat 2, fiber 2, carbs 4, protein 7

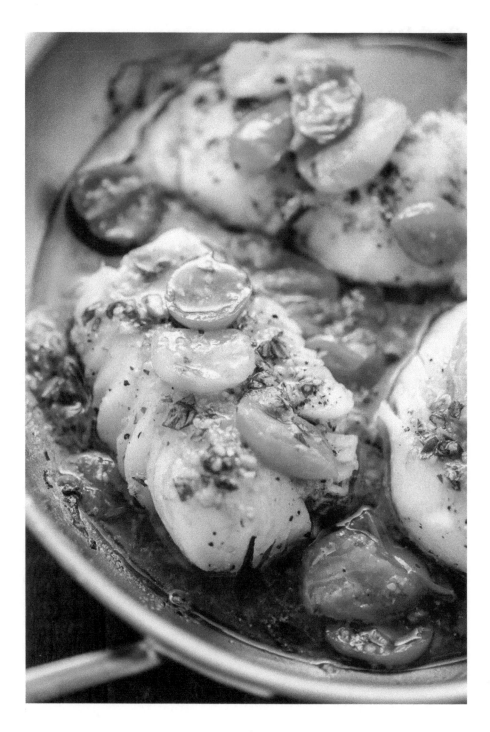

Chili Shrimp and Zucchinis

Prep Time:
5 minutes
Cook Time:
8 minutes
Serve: 4

Ingredients:

- 1 pound shrimp, peeled and deveined
- 2 tablespoons avocado oil
- 2 zucchinis, sliced
- Juice of 1 lime
- A pinch of salt and black pepper
- 2 red chilies, chopped
- 3 garlic cloves, minced
- 1 tablespoon balsamic vinegar

Directions:

1.Heat a pan with the oil over medium-high heat, add the shrimp, garlic and the chilies and cook for 3 minutes.

2.Add the rest of the ingredients, toss, cook everything for 5 minutes more, divide between plates and serve.

Nutrition: calories 211, fat 5, fiber 2, carbs 11, protein 15

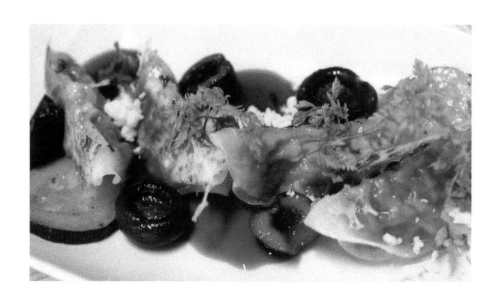

Lemon Scallops

Prep Time:
10 minutes
Cook Time:
10 minutes
Serve: 4

Ingredients:

- 2 tablespoons olive oil
- 1 pound sea scallops
- ½ teaspoon rosemary, dried
- ½ cup veggie stock
- 2 garlic cloves, minced
- Juice of ½ lemon

Directions:

1.Heat a pan with the oil over medium-high heat, add the garlic, the scallops and the other ingredients, cook everything for 10 minutes, divide into bowls and serve.

Nutrition: calories 170, fat 5, fiber 2, carbs 8, protein 10

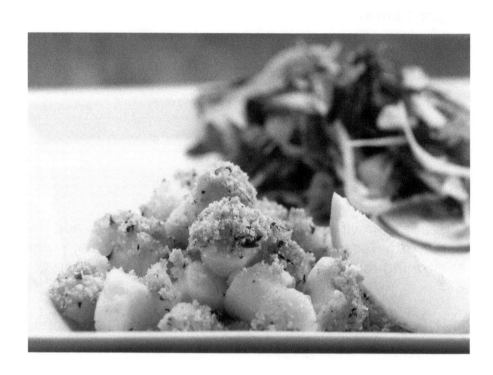

Crab and Shrimp Salad

Prep Time:
5 minutes
Cook Time:
0 minutes
Serve: 4

Ingredients:

- 1 cup canned crab meat, drained
- 1 pound shrimp, peeled, deveined and cooked
- 1 cup cherry tomatoes, halved
- 1 cucumber, sliced
- 2 cups baby arugula
- 2 tablespoons avocado oil
- 1 tablespoon chives, chopped
- 1 tablespoon lemon juice
- A pinch of salt and black pepper

Directions:

1.In a bowl, combine the shrimp with the crab meat and the other ingredients, toss and serve.

Nutrition: calories 203, fat 12, fiber 6, carbs 12, protein 9

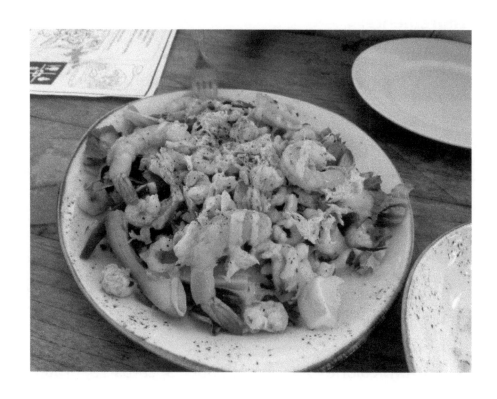

Salmon with Zucchinis and Tomatoes

Prep Time:
10 minutes
Cook Time:
30 minutes
Serve: 4

Ingredients:

- 4 salmon fillets, boneless
- 2 tablespoons avocado oil
- 2 tablespoons sweet paprika
- 2 zucchinis, sliced
- 2 tomatoes, cut into wedges
- ¼ teaspoon red pepper flakes, crushed
- A pinch of sea salt and black pepper
- 4 garlic cloves, minced

Directions:

1.In a roasting pan, combine the salmon with the oil and the other ingredients, toss gently and cook at 370 degrees F for 30 minutes.

2.Divide everything between plates and serve.

Nutrition: calories 210, fat 2, fiber 4, carbs 13, protein 10

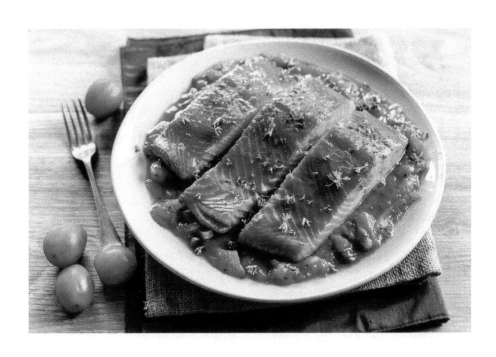

Shrimp and Mango Salad

Prep Time:
5 minutes
Cook Time:
0 minutes
Serve: 4

Ingredients:

- 1 pound shrimp, cooked, peeled and deveined
- 2 mangoes, peeled and cubed
- 3 scallions, chopped
- 1 cup baby spinach
- 1 cup baby arugula
- 1 jalapeno, chopped
- 2 tablespoons olive oil
- 1 tablespoon lime juice
- A pinch of salt and black pepper

Directions:

1.In a bowl, combine the shrimp with the mango, scallions and the other ingredients, toss and serve.

Nutrition: calories 210, fat 2, fiber 3, carbs 13, protein 8

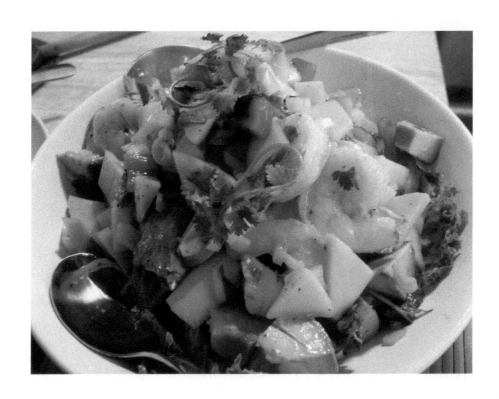

Creamy Cod Bowls

Prep Time:
5 minutes
Cook Time:
20 minutes
Serve: 4

Ingredients:

- 2 tablespoons olive oil
- 1 pound cod fillets, boneless and cubed
- 2 spring onions, chopped
- 2 garlic cloves, minced
- 1 cup coconut cream
- ¼ cup chives, chopped
- A pinch of salt and black pepper
- 2 tablespoons Dijon mustard

Directions:

1.Heat a pan with the oil over medium heat, add the garlic and the onions and sauté for 5 minutes.

2.Add the fish and the other ingredients, toss, cook over medium heat for 15 minutes more, divide into bowls.

Nutrition: calories 211, fat 5, fiber 5, carbs 6, protein 15

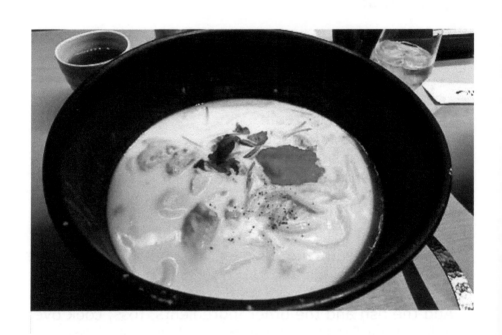

58

Trout and Cilantro Sauce

Prep Time:
5 minutes
Cook Time:
15 minutes
Serve: 4

Ingredients:

- 4 trout fillets, boneless
- 2 tablespoons avocado oil
- 1 cup cilantro, chopped
- 2 tablespoons lemon juice
- ½ cup coconut cream
- 1 tablespoon walnuts, chopped
- A pinch of salt and black pepper
- 3 teaspoons lemon zest, grated

Directions:

1.In a blender, combine the cilantro with the cream and the other ingredients except the fish and the oil and pulse well.

2.Heat a pan with the oil over medium heat, add the fish and cook for 4 minutes on each side.

3.Add the cilantro sauce, toss gently and cook over medium heat for 7 minutes more.

4.Divide the mix between plates and serve.

Nutrition: calories 212, fat 14.6, fiber 1.3, carbs 2.9, protein 18

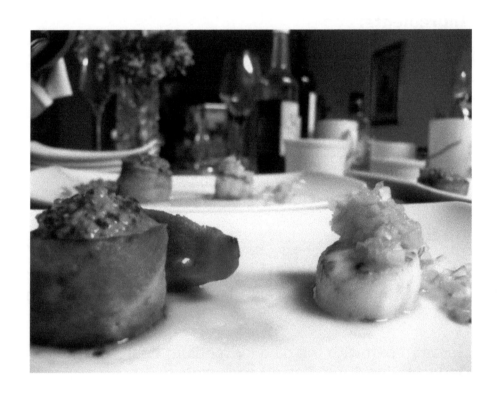

Basil Tilapia

Prep Time:
5 minutes
Cook Time:
12 minutes
Serve: 4

Ingredients:

- 4 tilapia fillets, boneless
- 2 tablespoons olive oil
- 2 tablespoons lemon juice
- 1 teaspoon basil, dried
- 1 tablespoon cilantro, chopped

Directions:

1.Heat a pan with the oil over medium heat, add the fish and cook for 5 minutes on each side.

2.Add the rest of the ingredients, toss gently, cook for 2 minutes more, divide between plates and serve.

Nutrition: calories 201, fat 8.6, fiber 0, carbs 0.2, protein 31.6

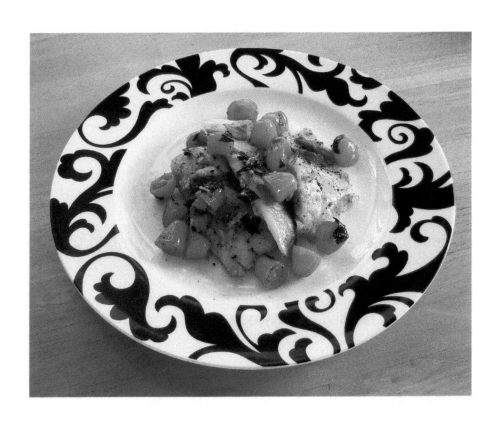

Mustard Salmon Mix

Prep Time:
5 minutes
Cook Time:
14 minutes
Serve: 4

Ingredients:

- 4 salmon fillets, boneless
- ½ teaspoon mustard seeds
- ½ cup mustard
- 2 tablespoons olive oil
- 4 scallions, chopped
- Salt and black pepper to the taste
- 2 green chilies, chopped
- ¼ teaspoon cumin, ground
- ¼ cup parsley, chopped

Directions:

1.Heat a pot with the oil over medium heat, add the scallions and the chilies and cook for 2 minutes.

2.Add the fish and cook for 4 minutes on each side.

3.Add the remaining ingredients, toss, cook everything for 4 more minutes, divide between plates and serve.

Nutrition: calories 397, fat 23.9, fiber 3.5, carbs 8,5, protein 40

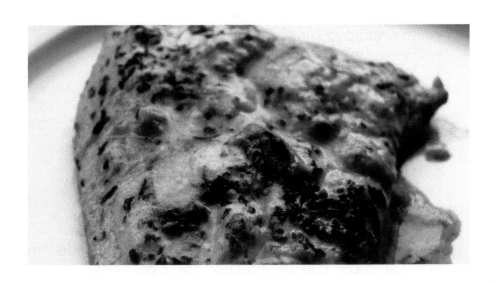

Shrimp and Cauliflower Mix

Prep Time:
10 minutes
Cook Time:
10 minutes
Serve: 4

Ingredients:

- 2 tablespoons olive oil
- 1 pound shrimp, peeled and deveined
- 1 cup cauliflower florets
- 2 tablespoons lemon juice
- 2 tablespoons garlic, minced
- 1 teaspoon cumin, ground
- 1 teaspoon turmeric powder
- Salt and black pepper to the taste

Directions;

1.Heat a pan with the oil over medium-high heat, add the garlic and sauté for 2 minutes.

2.Add the shrimp and cook for 4 minutes more.

3.Add the remaining ingredients, toss, cook the mix for 4 minutes, divide between plates and serve

Nutrition: calories 200, fat 5.3, fiber 3, carbs 11, protein 6

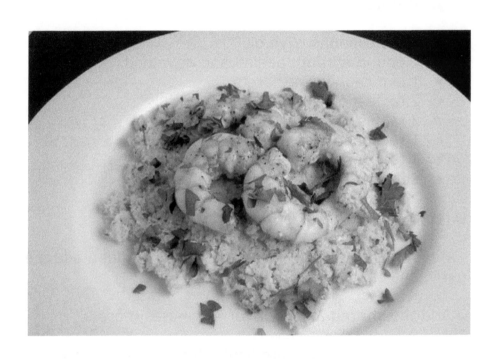

Salmon with Broccoli

Prep Time:
5 minutes
Cook Time:
15 minutes
Serve: 4

Ingredients:

- 4 salmon fillets, boneless
- 1 teaspoon coriander, ground
- 1 cup broccoli florets
- 2 tablespoons lemon juice
- 2 tablespoons avocado oil
- 1 tablespoon lemon zest, grated
- A pinch of salt and black pepper
- 2 tablespoons cilantro, chopped

Directions:

1.Heat a pan with the oil over medium heat, add the fish and cook for 4 minutes on each side.

2.Add the broccoli and the other ingredients, cook the mix for 7 more minutes, divide between plates and serve.

Nutrition: calories 210, fat 4.7, fiber 2, carbs 11, protein 17

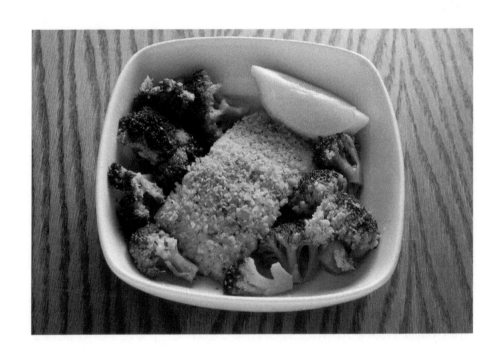

Salmon with Mushrooms

Prep Time:
10 minutes
Cook Time:
20 minutes
Serve: 4

Ingredients:

- 4 salmon fillets, boneless
- 2 tablespoons olive oil
- 1 cup mushrooms, sliced
- 3 green onions, chopped
- 1 tablespoon lime juice
- ¼ teaspoon nutmeg, ground
- ¼ cup almonds, toasted and chopped
- A pinch of salt

Directions:

1.Heat a pan with the oil over medium-high heat, add the green onions and sauté for 5 minutes.

2.Add the mushrooms and cook for 5 minutes more.

3.Add the fish and the other ingredients, cook it for 5 minutes on each side, divide between plates and serve.

Nutrition: calories 250, fat 10, fiber 3.3, carbs 7, protein 20

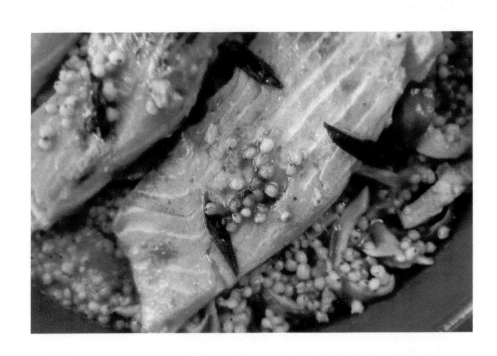

Shrimp with Rice

Prep Time:
10 minutes
Cook Time:
25 minutes
Serve: 4

Ingredients:

- 1 pound shrimp, peeled and deveined
- 1 cup black rice
- 2 cups chicken stock
- 4 scallions, chopped
- 1 teaspoon chili powder
- 1 teaspoon sweet paprika
- 2 tablespoons avocado oil
- A pinch of salt and black pepper

Directions:

1.Heat a pan with the oil over medium-high heat, add the scallions and sauté for 5 minutes.

2.Add the rice and the other ingredients except the shrimp, and cook the mix for 15 minutes.

3.Add the shrimp, cook everything for another 5 minutes, divide into bowls and serve.

Nutrition: calories 240, fat 7, fiber 6, carbs 8, protein 14

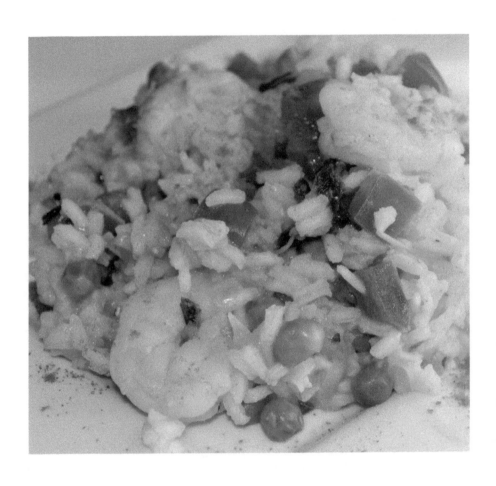

Dill Sea Bass

Prep Time:
5 minutes
Cook Time:
12 minutes
Serve: 4

Ingredients:

- 4 sea bass fillets, boneless
- 2 tablespoons olive oil
- 3 spring onions, chopped
- 2 tablespoons lemon juice
- Salt and black pepper to the taste
- 2 tablespoons dill, chopped

Directions:

1.Heat a pan with the oil over medium heat, add the onions and sauté for 2 minutes.

2.Add the fish and the other ingredients, cook everything for 5 minutes on each side, divide the mix between plates.

Nutrition: calories 214, fat 12, fiber 4, carbs 7, protein 17

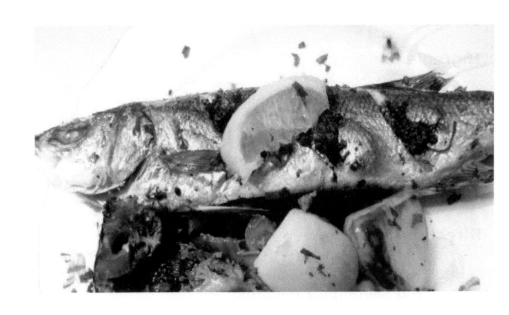

Trout with Tomato Sauce

Prep Time:
4 minutes
Cook Time:
15 minutes
Serve: 4

Ingredients:

- 4 trout fillets, boneless
- 2 spring onions, chopped
- 2 tablespoons olive oil
- 1 cup tomatoes, peeled and crushed
- ¼ cup coconut cream
- 1 tablespoon chives, chopped
- A pinch of salt and black pepper

Directions:

1.Heat a pan with the oil over medium heat, add the spring onions, tomatoes and the cream and cook for 5 minutes.

2.Add the fish and the rest of the ingredients, toss, cook everything for 10 minutes more, divide between plates.

Nutrition: calories 200, fat 5, fiber 6, carbs 12, protein 12

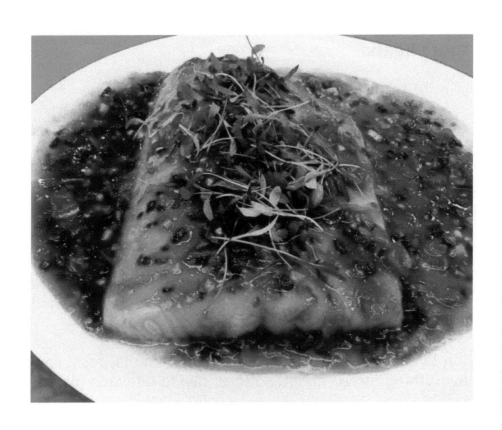

Breakfast Avocado and Tuna Balls

Prep Time:
5 minutes
Serve: 4

Ingredients:

- 1 can tuna
- 1 avocado, pitted and peeled
- 1/2 cup onion, chopped
- 1/2 teaspoon dried dill
- 3 ounces sunflower seed
- 1/2 teaspoon freshly ground black pepper
- 1/2 teaspoon smoked paprika
- Salt, to taste

Directions:

1.Add all ingredients in a mixing dish and mix thoroughly. Roll the mixture into 8 balls. Serve properly chilled and enjoy!

Nutrition: Calories 316, Protein 17.4g Protein 24: 4g, Carbs 5.9g, Sugar 1.4g

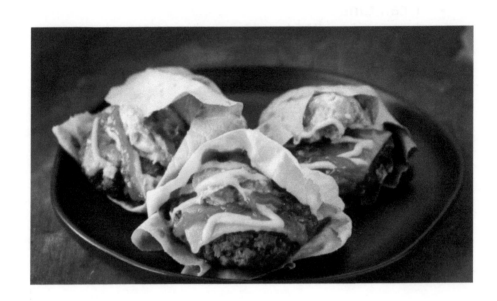

Smoked Tilapia Pie

Prep Time:
45 minutes
Serve: 6

Ingredients:

For the Crust:
- 3 tablespoons flaxseed meal
- 1/2 teaspoon baking powder
- 2 teaspoons ground psyllium husk powder
- 1/2 teaspoon kosher salt
- 1/2 teaspoon baking soda
- 1 cup almond flour
- 1/2 stick butter
- 2 tablespoons water
- 2 eggs

For the Filling:
- 1 teaspoon dried rosemary
- 1 ½ cups Cheddar cheese, shredded
- ½ teaspoon dried basil
- ½ cup mayonnaise
- 2 eggs
- ½ cup sour cream
- 10 ounces smoked tilapia, chopped
- Salt and ground black pepper, to taste
- 1 teaspoon Dijon mustard

Directions:

1.Beforehand, heat your oven to 3600F. Add all the crust ingredients in your food processor and mix. Line the baking pan with parchment paper and press the mixture into it.

2.Put the crust in the middle of the preheated oven and bake for approximately 13 minutes. Then, mix all the ingredients for the filling. Spread the mixture over the pie crust.

3.Bake for additional 30 minutes or until the pie is golden at the sides.

Nutrition: Calories 416, Protein 19.5g, Fat 34.2g, Carbs 5.5g, Sugar 1.7g

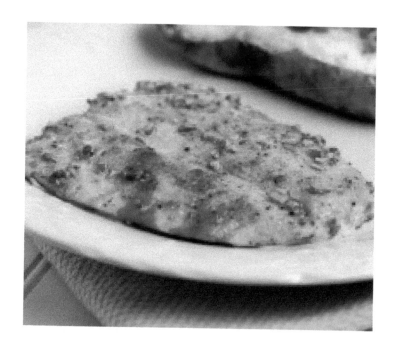

Spring Shrimp Salad

Prep Time:
10 minutes
Serve: 6

Ingredients:

- ½ teaspoon freshly ground black pepper
- 1 tablespoon wine vinegar
- 4 spring onions, chopped
- ½ cup sour cream
- ½ teaspoon yellow mustard
- 1 ½ cups radishes, sliced
- ½ cup mayonnaise
- 1 medium-sized lime, cut into wedges
- 1 tablespoon hot sauce
- 2 cucumbers, sliced
- 1 tablespoon Marsala wine
- 2 pounds shrimp

Directions:

1.Pour lime wedges and salt into a large pot; Boil over high heat.

2.After this, peel and devein the shrimp. Pour the shrimp and cook for 2 to 3 minutes until they are no longer transparent.

3.Drain and rinse the shrimp under running water. Then, peel your shrimp.

4.Put the remaining ingredients into a mixing dish and mix thoroughly. Add the shrimp and stir gently to mix evenly.

5.Place in the refrigerator until it is chill and ready to serve.

Nutrition: Calories 209, Protein 20.2g, Fat 9.5g, Carbs 6.8g, Sugar 2.1g

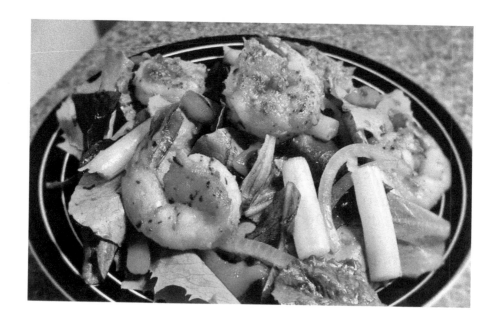

Salmon with Pine Nuts Sauce and Sautéed Brussels Sprouts

Prep Time:
25 minutes
Serve: 4

Ingredients:

- ½ pounds Brussels sprouts
- 1 tablespoon lime juice
- ½ cup chicken broth
- 1/3 cup fresh cilantro
- 1 pound salmon
- 1/3 cup pine nuts, chopped
- Sea salt and freshly ground black pepper, to taste
  1/4 cup olive oil
- 2 garlic cloves, crushed
- 1 teaspoon dried marjoram
- 1 medium-sized tomato, cut into slices

Directions:

1.Rub black pepper, salt and marjoram on the salmon on all sides; set aside.

2.Now, beat pine nuts, lemon juice, cilantro, olive oil, garlic in your food processor until it becomes a smooth paste.

3.Heat a nonstick skillet over moderately high heat. Spritz the base of the skillet with a nonstick cooking spray and fry the salmon on each side for 2 to 4 minutes; reserve.

4.In the same skillet, place Brussels sprouts and chicken broth; sauté for 4 to 6 minutes or until Brussels sprouts are as tender as you want; reserve.

5.In the same skillet, sear tomato slices for 2 minutes on each side.

6.Serve warm salmon with cilantro sauce and tomato slice topping, garnished with sautéed Brussels sprouts.

Nutrition: Calories 372, Protein 26.5g, Fat 27.8g, Carbs 5.6g, Sugar 2.6g

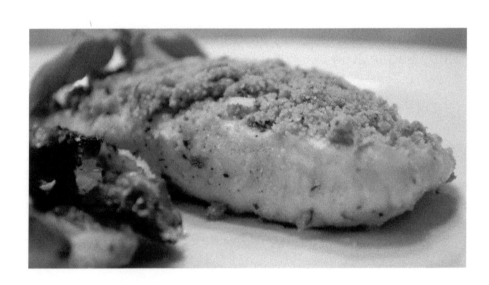

Aromatic Red Snapper Soup

Prep Time:
20 minutes
Serve: 4

Ingredients:

- ¼ cup fresh cilantro, chopped
- 1 pound red snapper, chopped
- 2 garlic cloves, minced
- 2 cups shellfish stock
- ¼ cup dry white wine
- Sea salt and ground black pepper, to taste
- 2 tomatoes, pureed
- 2 onions, finely chopped
- ½ stick butter, melted
- 2 rosemary sprigs, chopped
- 2 thyme sprigs, chopped
- ½ teaspoon dried dill weed
- 1 cup water

Directions:_

1.Preheat stockpot over moderate heat and melt the butter into the pot. Sauté the onions and garlic for 3 minutes or until aromatic.

2.Add the fresh cilantro and cook for 1 to 2 minutes more.

3.Add pureed tomatoes, fish, wine, water and stock; bring to a boil.

4.Reduce the heat and let it simmer until the fish is properly cooked about 15 minutes.

5.Add the remaining seasonings and serve warm.

Nutrition: Calories 316, Protein 32.7g, Fat 14.3g, Carbs 6.6g, Sugar 2.1g

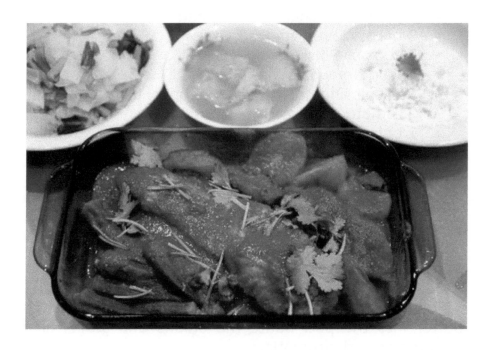

Easy Fried Tiger Prawns

Prep Time:
10 minutes
Serve: 4

Ingredients:

- 1 teaspoon dried rosemary
- 2 tablespoons dry sherry
- ½ stick butter, at room temperature
- ½ teaspoon mustard seeds
- 1 ½ tablespoons fresh lime juice
- 1 tablespoon garlic paste
- 1 ½ pounds tiger prawns, peeled and deveined
- 1 teaspoon red pepper flakes, crushed
- Salt and ground black pepper, to taste

Directions:

1. Place a mustard seed, dry sherry, lime juice, flakes, rosemary, garlic paste and red pepper in a mixing bowl and mix thoroughly.

2. Add the prawns to the mixture in the mixing dish and leave to marinate for 1 hour in the refrigerator.

3. Preheat skillet over medium-high heat and melt the butter in it. Dispose of the marinade and fry prawns for 3 to 5 minutes turning once or twice.

4. Season with salt and pepper to taste.

Nutrition: Calories 294, Protein 34.6g, Fat 14.3g, Carbs 3.6g, Sugar 0.1g

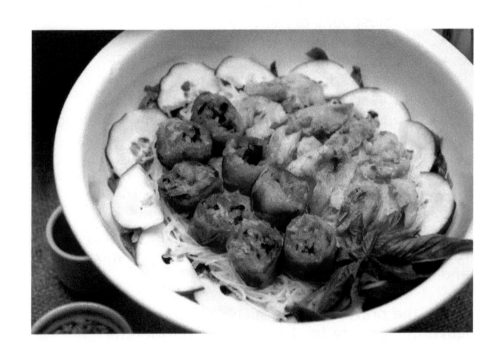

Saucy Chilean Sea Bass with Dijon Sauce

Prep Time:
15 minutes
Serve: 4

Ingredients:

- 1 cup scallions, chopped
- ½ cup dry sherry wine
- ½ teaspoon paprika
- 1 teaspoon Dijon mustard
- 2 cloves garlic, minced
- 1 pound wild Chilean sea bass, cubed
- ¼ teaspoon ground black pepper
- 1 tablespoon avocado oil
- 1 cup double cream
- 2 Poblano pepper, chopped
- Sea salt, to taste

Directions:

1.Toss the fish, garlic, peppers, salt, wine, paprika and scallion in a mixing bowl. Leave in the refrigerator for 2 hours to marinate.

2.Warm avocado oil in a cast-iron skillet over a medium heat.

3.Cook the fish and marinade until it is thoroughly cooked, about 5 minutes; reserve cooked fish.

4.In the same skillet, add the double cream, ground black pepper and Dijon mustard.

5.Bring to a boil, and then, reduce the heat.
6.Continue cooking until everything is heated through, approximately 3 minutes.

7.Add the fish back to the skillet, remove from heat and serve immediately.

Nutrition: Calories 228, Protein 13.7g, Fat 13g, Carbs 6.5g, Sugar 2.1g

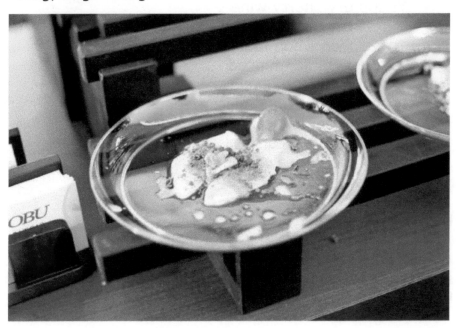

Two-Cheese and Smoked Salmon Dip

Prep Time:
10 minutes
Serve: 10

Ingredients:

- 10 ounces smoked salmon, chopped
- 5 ounces Cottage cheese
- 5 ounces Feta cheese
- 4 hard-boiled egg yolks, finely chopped
- Salt and freshly ground black pepper, to your liking
- 1/2 teaspoon smoked paprika
- 1/4 cup fresh chives, chopped

Directions:

1.Place all ingredients, except for chopped chives into a mixing dish.

2.Stir well until the mixture is evenly mixed.

3.Put in a mound on a dish.

4.Garnish with fresh chopped chives and serve well-chilled.

Nutrition: Calories 109, Protein11.4g, Fat 6.3g, Carbs 1.3g, Sugar 0.8g

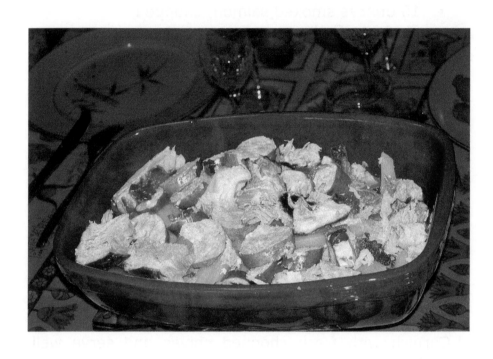

Halibut Steaks for Two

Prep Time:
35 minutes
Serve: 2

Ingredients:

- 1 teaspoon dry thyme
- 1/3 cup fresh cilantro, chopped
- 1/3 cup fresh lime juice
- 2 teaspoons olive oil
- 1/3 teaspoon salt
- 2 halibut steaks
- 1/3 teaspoon pepper
- 1 teaspoon garlic, finely minced
- 1 teaspoon dry dill weed

Directions:

1.In a mixing bowl, combine fresh lime juice with olive oil, salt, pepper, dill, thyme and garlic. Add halibut steak and let it marinate about 20 minutes.

2.Now, grill your fish steaks approximately 13 minutes, turning once or twice; make sure to baste them with the reserved marinade.

3.Garnish with fresh cilantro leaves. Serve warm with your favorite salad.

Nutrition: Calories 308, Protein 46.5g, Fat 10.9g, Carbs 2g, Sugar 0.2g

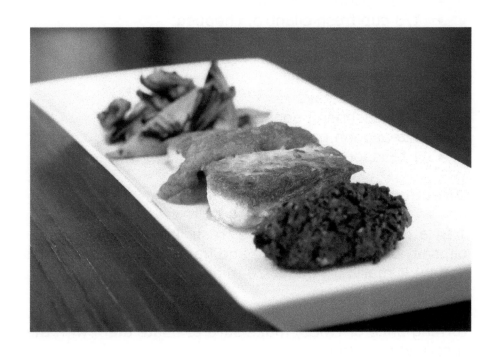

Tuna and Avocado Salad with Mayo Dressing

Prep Time:
5 minutes
Serve: 4

Ingredients:

- 1 teaspoon deli mustard
- 1/2 cup Kalamata olives, pitted and sliced
- 2 bell peppers, deveined and sliced
- 2 cans tuna chunks in spring water
- 1 head arugula
- 1 red onion, chopped
- 1 avocado, pitted, peeled and diced
- Salt and ground black pepper, to taste
- 2 tablespoons fresh lime juice
- 1 cup cherry tomatoes, halved or quartered
- 1/4 cup mayonnaise

Directions:

1.Combine tuna, avocado, bell peppers, cherry tomato, arugula and onion in a salad bowl.

2.In a small mixing bowl, whisk the mayonnaise with mustard, salt, pepper and lime juice. Dress the salad and gently toss to combine.

3.Top with Kalamata olives and serve well-chilled.

Nutrition: Calories 244, Protein 23.4g, Fat 12.7g, Carbs 5.3g, Sugar 2.8g

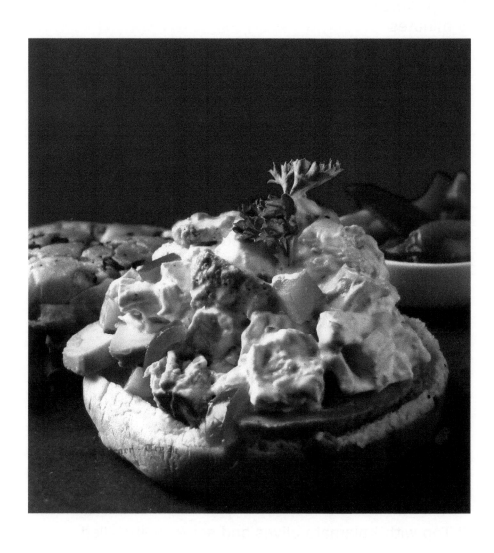

Pan-Seared Fish Fillets with Mesclun Salad

Prep Time:
15 minutes
Serve: 4

Ingredients:

- 4 white fish fillets
- 1 tablespoon butter, softened
- 2 tablespoons fresh coriander, chopped
- 2 garlic cloves, minced
- 2 tablespoons fresh lime juice
- Salt and ground black pepper, to taste
- 2 tablespoons fresh chives, chopped

For Mesclun Salad:
- Salt and ground black pepper, to your liking
- 1 cup arugula
- 1 head Romaine lettuce
- ¼ cup extra-virgin olive oil
- 2 tablespoons basil, chiffonade
- 1 cup chicory
- 2 tablespoons dandelion
- ½ cup apple cider vinegar

Directions:

1.Toss white fish fillets with garlic, salt, lime juice, chives, pepper, and coriander; permit it to marinate at least 1 hour in the refrigerator.

2.Dissolve the butter in a pan over a normal heat; sear the fish fillets on each side for about 4 minutes. Now, use the marinade as a basting sauce.

3.Meanwhile, place Romaine lettuce, arugula, chicory, basil and dandelion in a salad container.

4.Then, make a dressing for your salad by whisking the remaining ingredients. Now, dress the salad and serve with warm fish fillets. Bon appétit!

Nutrition: Calories 425, Protein 38.3g, Fat 27.2g, Carbs 6.1g, Sugar 4.1g

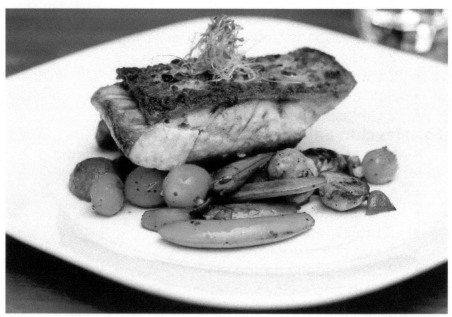

Mediterranean-Style Snapper Salad

Prep Time:
15 minutes
Serve: 4

Ingredients:

- 4 cups baby spinach
- 4 snapper fillets
- 2 tablespoons butter, melted
- 12 grape tomatoes, halved
- ½ cup ripe olives, pitted and sliced
- 2 shallots, thinly sliced
- 1 teaspoon ground sumac
- Sea salt and ground black pepper, to taste
- 6 ounces Halloumi cheese, crumbled

For the Vinaigrette:
- 1 teaspoon red pepper flakes, crushed
- 2 tablespoons fresh mint, finely chopped
- 1/2 tablespoon brown mustard
- 1 clove garlic, smashed
- Sea salt and ground black pepper, to taste
- 1/3 cup extra-virgin olive oil
- 1 lemon, juiced and zested
- 1 teaspoon dried oregano

Directions:

1.Place the fish fillets on a clean board and spray both sides with salt, pepper and sumac.

2.Then, warm the butter in a pan that is preheated over a normal flame. Fry the fish for about 5 minutes on each side.

3.In a nice salad container, tomatoes, toss baby spinach, shallots, cheese and olives. Then top with chopped fish.

4.Thoroughly merge all ingredients for the vinaigrette in your blender. Then, dress the salad and serve well-chilled.

Nutrition: Calories 507, Protein 24.4g, Fat 42.8g, Carbs 6g, Sugar 2.2g

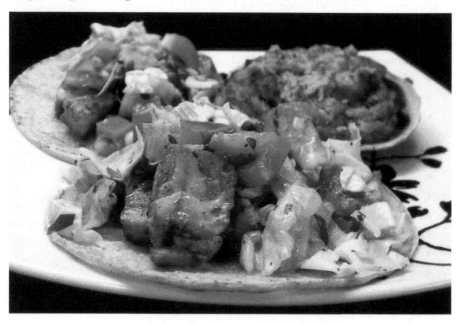

Prawn Cocktail Salad

Prep Time:
10 minutes
Serve: 6

Ingredients:

- 2 pounds prawns, peeled leaving tails intact
- ½ cup mayonnaise
- 1⊠ cup chopped fresh dill
- Sea salt and freshly ground black pepper, to taste
- 1 teaspoon deli mustard
- Juice from 1 fresh lemon
- ½ cup cucumber, chopped
- 1 cup scallions, chopped
- ½ head Romaine lettuce, torn into pieces

Directions:

1.Start a pot of salted water to a boil; Heat the prawns for 3 minutes. Drain and pour in a mixing bowl; permit them to cool completely.

2.Toss carefully with the remaining ingredients. Put it in the refrigerator until ready to serve.

Nutrition: Calories 196, Protein 21.4g, Fat 8.3g, Carbs 6.5g, Sugar 2.3g

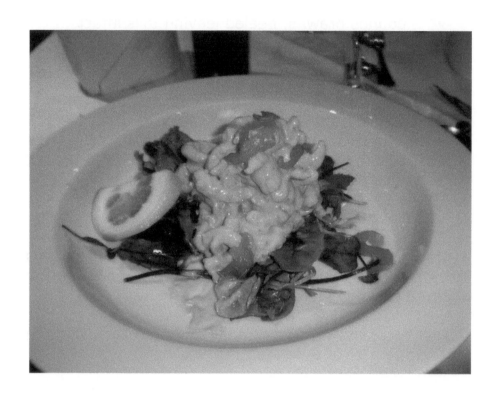

Halibut en Persillade

Prep Time:
20 minutes
Serve: 4

Ingredients:

- ½ cup scallions, sliced
- 2 cloves garlic, finely minced
- 1 ½ tablespoons olive oil
- 2 tablespoons fresh cilantro, chopped
- 4 halibut steaks
- 1 teaspoon garlic
- Salt and ground black pepper, to taste
- ¼ cup fresh parsley, finely chopped
- 3 tablespoons clam juice
- 1 tablespoon fresh lime juice
- 2 tablespoons coconut oil, at room temperature
- 1 tablespoon Worcestershire sauce
- ½ teaspoon fresh ginger, grated
- 1 tablespoon oyster sauce
- ½ fresh lemon, zested and juiced

Directions:

1.Heat the oil in a cast-iron skillet over a hot flame until it begins to smoke.

2.Fry halibut until golden brown, approximate time of 7 minutes. Turn and fry on the other side for an additional 4 minutes. Reserve.

3.Heat the scallions and garlic in pan drippings until tender. Include the remaining ingredients along with reserved halibut steaks, cover and heat for 5 minutes more.

105

4.Share among four plates.

5.Now, whisk the remaining ingredients to make Persillade sauce. Spoon over halibut steaks on the plates and enjoy.

Nutrition: Calories 273, Protein 22.6g, Fat 19.2g, Carbs 4.3g, Sugar 1.6g

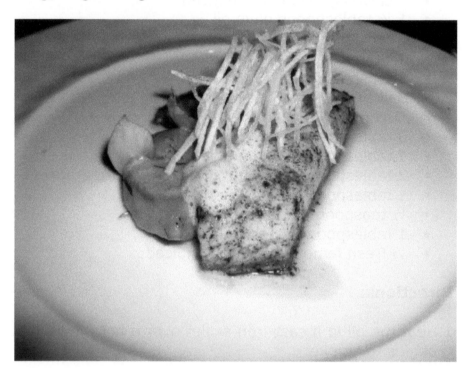

Hearty Pollock Chowder

Prep Time:
30 minutes
Serve: 4

Ingredients:

- 2 shallots, chopped
- 3 cups boiling water
- 3 teaspoons butter
- ¼ cup dry white wine
- 1 celery with leaves, chopped
- Sea salt and ground black pepper, to taste
- ½ cup full-fat milk
- 1 teaspoon Old Bay seasonings
- 1 ¼ pounds pollock fillets, skin removed
- ½ cup clam juice

Directions:

1.Slice pollock fillets into bite-sized pieces.

2.Warm the butter in a pan over an average-high flame. Heat the vegetables until they're softened. Season with pepper, salt, and Old Bay seasonings.

3.Mix in chopped fish and heat for 12 to 15 minutes more. Include the boiling water and clam juice. Now, pour in the white wine and milk.

4.Now, bring it to a boil. Decrease the heat and cook for an additional 15 minutes.

Nutrition: Calories 170, Protein 20g, Fat 5.8g, Carbs 5.7g, Sugar 2.2g

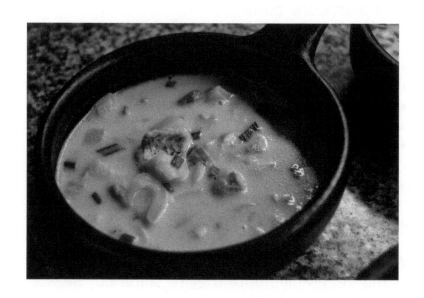

Lightning Source UK Ltd.
Milton Keynes UK
UKHW052040040621
384855UK00004BA/87